MAYR DIET

FOR BEGINNERS

A FUNDAMENTAL AND COMPLETE GUIDE FOR BEGINNERS TO LOSE WEIGHT FAST, BOOST YOUR METABOLISM, BURN EXCESS FAT WITH QUICK AND EASY TO MAKE RECIPES

BY

Dr. Jennifer Washington

&

Dr. Pamela Rogers

©COPYRIGHT

All Rights Reserved. Contents of this book may not be reproduced in any way or by any means without written consent of the publisher, with exception of brief excerpts in critical reviews and articles.

Table of contents

©COPYRIGHT 2
CHAPTER 1 5
INTRODUCTION 5
CHAPTER 2 6
WHAT TO DO & WHAT NOT TO DO WHILE ON THE MAYR DIET 6
CHAPTER 3 8
HOW THE MAYR DIET WILL ASSIST YOU TO LOSE WEIGHT 8
CHAPTER 4 9
IS THE MAYR METHOD DIET SAFE AND EFFECTIVE? 9
CHAPTER 5 10
HOW TO STAY MOTIVATED WHILE ON THE MAYR DIET 10
CHAPTER 6 11
STARTING YOUR DIET PLANS 11
MAYR DIETS 11
  SPICY GINGER SESAME ASIAN CUCUMBER SALAD 11
  SKINNY BANG BANG ZUCCHINI NOODLES MEAL PREP 13
  CHICKEN LO MEIN 15
  GUACAMOLE RECIPE 18
  HEALTHY CHICKEN PAD THAI 20
  SHRIMP WITH ZUCCHINI 23
  HUMMUS PASTA 25
  ZUCCHINI LASAGNA ROLL-UPS 27
  ZUCCHINI FRITTERS WITH GARLIC HERB YOGURT SAUCE 29
  WARM WHITE BEAN & KALE SALAD 32
  CREAMY SHRIMP PASTA WITH CORN AND TOMATOES 33
  TOMATO SPINACH CHICKEN SPAGHETTI 35

FENNEL SALAD WITH CUCUMBER AND DILL	37
CABBAGE SALAD WITH CORN	38
SPINACH AND SUN-DRIED TOMATO ZOODLES	39
CLASSIC POTATO PANCAKES	41
ZUCCHINI NOODLES WITH AVOCADO SAUCE	43
EASY CREAMY CHICKEN PICCATA	44
SWEET AND SOUR CUCUMBER NOODLES	46
ROASTED BROCCOLI QUINOA SALAD	48
HONEY GARLIC ROASTED CARROTS	50
KALE SALAD	51
GARLIC HERB ROASTED POTATOES CARROTS AND GREEN BEANS	52
ROASTED CAULIFLOWER STEAKS	54
HOT TURKEY AND CHEESE PARTY ROLLS	56
CONCLUSION	58

CHAPTER 1

INTRODUCTION

According to Dr. Maximilian Schubert, the medical director of VivaMayr, an Austrian health facility that supports the diet, said that while some modifications have been made in the past century, the Mayr diet still adheres to its roots. The main idea behind this is that they will have a holistic approach to health if individuals have a healthy gut system and a healthy digestive system.

For two weeks, you will feel like a totally different individual. You're going to feel more energetic; your skin is glowing, you're going to sleep better, you're going to think more clearly, you're going to lose weight. What's more, you should also get down with things such as food intolerances if there are problems - you should, too.

They are also starting to see a noticeable improvement. With time, they might even be able, permanently, to vanish. Viva Mayr helps through a signature detox that includes some spa treatments, mental health sessions, & a thorough diet & fitness revamp.

CHAPTER 2

WHAT TO DO & WHAT NOT TO DO WHILE ON THE MAYR DIET

- One small cup of good coffee a day is okay.
- Ensure you make breakfast the biggest meal of your day, reasonable for lunch, and very small and light for dinner. Eat your dinner as early as possible, starting at 5 p.m. (Viva Mayr dinner time)
- Practice food combining, as far as possible. So, eat vegetable carbohydrates or vegetable proteins, but try to avoid mixing protein and carbohydrates in the same meal.
- Avoid eating snacks, in-between meals.
- Smoothies in small quantities are okay.
- Just keep chewing. The more you chew your meals, the more easily digestible you make them. Digestion, remember, begins with saliva in the mouth.
- Raw food is good, providing you chew correctly.
- Eat at a table at all times, without distractions. So, there's no reading, no watching TV, no working at your desk, no surfing the internet.
- Keep your cold liquids separate from your meals.

- Before you eat, smell your food. Your brain will understand what you're about to eat and will instruct your digestive system to alert the right enzymes and acids needed to deal with the load that comes in.

CHAPTER 3

HOW THE MAYR DIET WILL ASSIST YOU TO LOSE WEIGHT

Yes! The Mayr diet will assist you to lose weight in as much as you adhere strictly to the diet procedures.

Mayr Method specialists accept as true that the vital to decent health besides ideal weight loss is through good and clean diet. Later, the Mayr diet places a robust importance on including diets which soothes and improve digestion.

Mayr Method has its derivation in traditional viewpoint & speaks the worth of mindful consumption

CHAPTER 4

IS THE MAYR METHOD DIET SAFE AND EFFECTIVE?

In as much as you don't brutally curb calories or nutriments once you follow the Mayr Method diet, this method of food consumption can be very safe and more effective.

CHAPTER 5

HOW TO STAY MOTIVATED WHILE ON THE MAYR DIET

It is always half the fight to stay motivated for weight loss, as your expectations will get in the way of maintaining your ideal weight.

See a doctor regarding potential mental health therapies that can relieve you or improve your mood and level of motivation during weight loss if you suffer from chronic stress, anxiety, or depression that influences eating habits and your calorie consumption.

CHAPTER 6

STARTING YOUR DIET PLANS

MAYR DIETS

SPICY GINGER SESAME ASIAN CUCUMBER SALAD

Recipes

- Two medium cucumbers, sliced thin into rounds or ribbons using a spiralizer or sharp knife
- fine sea salt
- One tablespoon finely minced jalapeño pepper (optional)
- 1/4 cup thinly sliced red onion
- One tablespoon toasted sesame seed
- Two tablespoons fresh cilantro, roughly chopped

Procedures

- Place in a colander the thinly sliced cucumbers and sprinkle with a few pinches of sea salt, allowing them to sit while preparing the other ingredients. (This is so the cucumber water does not water-down the dressing).

- Make the dressing whilst the cucumbers are sitting. In a small clean bowl, add all of the ingredients. Whisk to combine well.
- Rinse the cucumbers once you are ready to assemble the salad and pat it dry with paper towels or a clean kitchen towel. Transfer them to a large bowl of salad.

Put the red onions, the minced jalapeño, half the sesame seeds, and half the cilantro in the mixture. To combine all, pour the dressing over the top of the salad and toss gently. Sprinkle on top with the remaining sesame seeds and the rest of the cilantro. Chill until it's ready for serving. Enjoy! Enjoy!

SKINNY BANG BANG ZUCCHINI NOODLES MEAL PREP

Recipes:

- Four medium zucchini spiralized
- 1 tbsp of olive oil

Sauce

- 1/4 cup + 2 tbsp of fat-free plain Greek yogurt
- 1/4 cup + 2 tbsp of light mayonnaise
- 1/4 cup + 2 tbsp of Thai sweet chili sauce
- 1 1/2 tbsp of honey
- 1 1/2 tsp of sriracha sauce
- 2 tsps. of lime juice

Procedures

- Cook them first on the stove if you are using any proteins, and set aside.
- Add olive oil to a large skillet and bring to medium-high heat to cook the zucchini. Stir in the zucchini noodles once the oil is hot. Cook until the water and zucchini have just been cooked (tender but still crisp).
- Switch the heat off. Drain zucchini noodles. Allow noodles to rest and drain away any other release of water for about 10 minutes.

- Place all the recipes for the sauce in a large bowl. Mix until smooth with a whisk. Taste as needed and adjust. In 4 small containers, pour sauce. Once everything has cooled, mix zucchini noodles with your proteins and add them to meal prep containers.
- Store it well in the refrigerator & consume it within three days.
- To prepare for the day, heat the noodles. Drain any water from the noodles that may be released. Toss in the dressing sauce (sauce can be used hot or cold; I prefer to keep it cold & mix it well with the hot noodles).

CHICKEN LO MEIN

Recipes:

For Sauce

- 1 tbsp of brown sugar packed
- 2 tbsp of soy sauce low sodium
- 2 tbsp of dark soy sauce
- 1 tbsp of oyster sauce
- 1 tsp of hoisin sauce
- 1 tsp of ground black pepper
- 1 tsp of sesame oil

For Chicken

- 1 lb of chicken breasts skinless & boneless, cut into small pieces
- 2 tbsp of soy sauce
- 1 tsp of fresh ginger minced
- Three cloves of garlic minced
- 2 tbsp olive oil

For Veggies

- 2 tbsp olive oil
- 2 cups shiitake mushrooms sliced
- 1 cup Chinese cabbage shredded

- 1 cup carrots julienned
- One large onion chopped

Other

- 16 oz ramen noodles or any other Asian style noodles
- Three green onions chopped

Procedures

- According to package directions, cook the noodles. Drain it yourself and set it aside.
- Whisk the sauce ingredients all together in a small bowl, then set aside.
- Toss the chicken and the soy sauce, ginger, and garlic together in another medium-sized bowl.
- In a large wok, heat up the olive oil well. Before adding the chicken to it, your wok should be pretty and hot. Cook for about five minutes or until the chicken begins to brown and is no longer pink inside. Add the seasoned chicken. Transfer the chicken and set it aside on a plate.
- Then add the shiitake mushrooms, cabbage, carrots & onion to the wok and add the other two tablespoons of olive oil to the wok. Cook while tossing around for a minute.

- Add the chicken to the wok again. Add the cooked noodles, the sauce, and toss it all together. Turn the heat off.
- Garnish with green onions and proceed to serve.

GUACAMOLE RECIPE

Recipes:

- 1/4 cup of finely minced onion
- Three ripe Haas of avocados
- 1 1/2 tablespoons of fresh lime juice (or lemon juice)
- One big Plum or Roma tomato, deseeded & diced
- 1/4 cup of cilantro leaves & tender stems, chopped
- 1/2 teaspoon of ground cumin, optional
- 1/2 teaspoon of salt, or more
- 1 to 2 teaspoons of minced jalapeño or serrano pepper, with seeds & membrane removed, non-compulsory

Procedures:

- In a small clean bowl, add the diced onion, then cover with warm water, set aside for 5 minutes, and drain. The onions are "de-flamed" by this, making them less intense.
- Gently cut the avocados into half, & remove the pit lengthwise. Scoop the flesh out, then add it to a bowl.
- Use a clean fork to mash until creamy but still chunky, then add lime juice. Tomatoes, cilantro, cumin, drained de-flamed onions, salt, and diced peppers are mixed together (if using).

- Taste and adjust the guacamole with added salt, pepper, or lime juice. By moving the plastic wrap down onto the guacamole, serve immediately or cover with plastic wrap and refrigerate up to one day.

HEALTHY CHICKEN PAD THAI

Recipes:

- 5 oz of brown rice noodles
- Two tablespoons of olive oil
- 1 lb of chicken breasts pounded thinly
- 1 cup of red peppers sliced into thin pieces
- 2 cups of carrots sliced into thin pieces
- 1/2 cup of chopped onion
- One tablespoon of garlic minced
- 1 cup of Bean sprouts
- Two large eggs

For the Sauce:

- One tablespoon peanut butter
- Two tablespoons honey
- Two tablespoons lime juice
- 1.5 tablespoons rice wine vinegar
- ¼ cup of fish sauce
- ¼ cup of coconut aminos or a low sodium soy sauce

For Garnish:

- 1/4 cup green onions sliced thinly

- ⅓ cup peanuts crushed or chopped
- red pepper flakes (optional)
- lime wedges (optional)
- cilantro (optional)

Procedures:

- Cut the chicken into square 1-inch pieces. Gently heat the olive oil in a big clean pan over medium-high heat. Add the cubed chicken to the pan and cook for 12-15 minutes over medium-high heat until fully browned and cooked!
- Carry a clean pot of water to a boil during chicken cooking + cook rice noodles according to the instructions on the package.
- While cooking noodles/chicken, whisk the ingredients for the sauce together and set off to the side. Chop the veggies.
- Detach the chicken from the pan + put it aside in a large bowl once the chicken has cooked. Try to leave the pan with the oil.
- Add the peppers, carrots, garlic, and onion to the oil and sauté for 10 minutes, uncovered. Stir in the bean sprouts after ten minutes and cook for an additional two minutes.

- Push vegetables into the pan on one side of the pan + crack eggs. Scramble for about two minutes until the eggs are cooked.
- Stir veggie/egg mixture together. Take it out of the pan and set it aside with the chicken.
- Add the mixture of sauce to the empty pan (you don't need to clean the pan!) & bring to a low boil whilst constantly stirring for one minute. It should bubble and thicken the sauce slightly.
- In the saucepan, add the cooked veggies, cooked chicken, and cooked noodles and toss to combine.
- Garnish well with peanuts. Optional garnish: lime, green onions, cilantro.

SHRIMP WITH ZUCCHINI

Recipes:

- 2 tbsp. Of olive oil
- 450 gr. Of shrimp, peeled and deveined
- Three minced garlic cloves.
- 1/2 tsp. of chopped red pepper
- 2 tbsp. of lemon juice
- 1/2 tsp. of lemon zest
- 1/2 teaspoon of salt
- 1/4 tsp of ground black pepper
- Three medium zucchinis, spiralized
- 2 tbsp of grated Parmesan
- Two tablespoons of chopped parsley

Procedures:

- Carefully Heat a skillet over medium-high heat using oil.
- Then proceed to Add the shrimp, black pepper, sea salt, & red pepper.
- Proceed to cook until shrimp are pink, for up to five minutes.
- Add the lemon zest, lemon juice & garlic.

- Add the spiralized zucchini noodles & Parmesan, and mix very well.
- It can also be garnished with parsley for a lovely decoration!

HUMMUS PASTA

Recipes:

- Two tablespoons olive oil
- One medium onion sliced
- Two garlic cloves sliced
- 1 cup spinach
- 1 cup plain hummus
- 1 pound spaghetti pasta
- Juice of 1 lemon + zest
- ¼ cup of freshly chopped basil plus more for serving
- Pinch of crushed red pepper

Procedures:

- Over high heat, bring a large pot of salted water to a low boil. Add the pasta & cook following the package instructions until al dente. Move aside one cup of pasta cooking water, then drain the pasta and put it back in the pot to keep warm.
- Gently heat the olive oil in a clean big skillet over medium heat. Add the onions and cook for 5-7 minutes or until they are soft and fragrant. Add the garlic & cook until fragrant or for 30 seconds. Add the spinach & cook until it is slightly wilted, or 1 minute.

- Add the hummus, ½ cup of pasta cooking water, lemon juice, and lemon zest, and stir until the sauce is creamy. Put extra pasta water, as needed, to thin the sauce a bit at a time.
- Transfer to the skillet the cooked pasta, turn off the heat, and toss it all together. Add basil and crushed red pepper to top.
- If desired, serve immediately with parmesan cheese or basil.

ZUCCHINI LASAGNA ROLL-UPS

Recipes:

- Six big zucchinis
- 1 (16-oz.) container of ricotta
- 3/4 c. freshly grated Parmesan, divided
- Two big eggs
- 1/2 tsp. of garlic powder
- Kosher salt
- Freshly ground pepper (black)
- 1 cup of marinara
- 1 cup of grated mozzarella

Procedures:

- Preheat the oven to 400 degrees. Lengthwise slice zucchini into 1/8 inches thick strips, then place strips on a baking sheet lined with a paper towel to drain.
- Make a mixture of ricotta: combine ricotta, 1/2 cup Parmesan cheese, eggs, and garlic powder in a small bowl, and season well with salt & pepper.
- Spread a thin layer of marinara on the bottom of a 9-inch by 13-inch baking dish. Spoon a thin layer of sauce on both slices of zucchini, spread the ricotta mixture on

top, and sprinkle with mozzarella. Roll up and place in a tightly packed baking dish.
- Sprinkle with another 1/4 cup of Parmesan cheese. Bake for up to 20 minutes, until the zucchini is tender and the cheese melts.

ZUCCHINI FRITTERS WITH GARLIC HERB YOGURT SAUCE

Garlic Herb Yogurt Sauce

- 1/2 cup of plain Greek or regular yogurt
- Two teaspoons of chopped parsley
- 1 Tablespoon of chopped fresh mint
- 2 Tablespoons of fresh lemon juice
- 1 Tablespoon of olive oil
- One teaspoon of honey
- One heaping teaspoon of minced garlic
- salt & fresh ground black pepper, to taste

Fritters

- 2 cups of shredded zucchini (2 small or one large zucchini)
- 1 cup of shredded sweet potato (1 small, peeled)
- 1/3 cup of finely chopped onion
- 1 and 1/2 teaspoons of salt
- Two big eggs
- One heaping teaspoon of minced garlic
- 2 Tablespoons of chopped parsley
- 2 Tablespoons of chopped fresh mint
- 1/2 teaspoon of freshly ground pepper black

- 1/3 cup of cornmeal
- 1 Tablespoon of cornstarch
- 1/3 cup of olive oil

Procedures:

- Create the yogurt sauce by whisking together all the ingredients for the yogurt sauce except the salt and pepper. Taste to taste, then add salt/pepper to taste. Cover and refrigerate until ready to serve.
- Make the fritters: In a large strainer, place the shredded zucchini, sweet potato, and onion. Put one teaspoon of salt on top and mix it with a large wooden spoon. To start draining some of the water out of the vegetables, press down with your hands. Let it sit for some time in the sink.
- Meanwhile, with paper towels or a clean dish towel, line a large bowl (easier to use a towel!). Place the mixture of vegetables in the bowl and top the dish towel with more paper towels or fold over. Start pressing down; you need as much liquid as possible to get out.
- As required, grab more paper towels or a new dish towel. Note: you can also simply wring the vegetables over the sink in the dishtowel. Simply keep, wringing! Let the vegetables sit for 45 minutes on the towels, then

press again. The goal is to remove as much moisture as possible. Otherwise, they'll be soggy fritters. How much water you wring out will amaze you!
- In a large bowl, whisk the eggs together. Whisk in the garlic, parsley, mint, remaining 1/2 teaspoon salt, and pepper beat. Fold in the vegetables and add the cornmeal and cornstarch until all is mixed together.
- Heat oil over medium-high heat in a skillet. Use a fork to scoop up about two tablespoons of the zucchini mixture when hot (I always eyeball the amount). The bottom of the bowl may have liquid pooling, so make sure you use a fork, so the excess liquid is not in your fritter.
- Top the hot skillet with the mixture and flatten it with a spatula. Repeat with a few more, making sure the skillet does not overcrowd. Cook until golden brown, each side for about 3 minutes. Transfer until finished to a paper towel-lined plate.
- Serve warm fritters and sauce with yogurt.

WARM WHITE BEAN & KALE SALAD

Recipes:

- Four slices of sourdough bread
- Olive oil
- Haven's Kitchen Herby Chimichurri
- One bunch of dinosaur kale, chopped
- Two 15oz cans of white beans, drained & rinsed
- ½ of red onion, thinly sliced

Procedures

- Make croutons: gently heat the oven to 400 degrees F. Have the bread cut into cubes. Toss the olive oil with a glug. Spread on a clean baking sheet and bake until crispy, for about 10 minutes. Remove from the oven and toss the croutons in a bowl with about half the Chimichurri pouch. Just set aside.
- Heat enough oil in a clean large skillet to coat the pan. Add the kale, and add the beans and the red onion when you see it start to wilt.
- Cut the heat and squeeze another ¼ pouch of Chimichurri in the pan once they're warm and stir. Toss to taste with croutons, more sauce, and salt.

CREAMY SHRIMP PASTA WITH CORN AND TOMATOES

Recipes:

- 8 ounces of linguine, spaghetti, or similar
- 1/2 cup of reserved pasta water
- Two tablespoons of butter, divided
- 1 lb. of shrimp, peeled & deveined (tail off or on, it's up to you)
- One teaspoon of salt, divided
- 1–2 cloves of garlic, minced
- 2 cups of cherry tomatoes, halved
- 2–3 ears of cooked or grilled fresh sweet corn, kernels cut off the cob
- 1 cup of fresh spinach, chopped
- a squeeze of lemon juice
- 1/2 - 3/4 cup of heavy cream
- fresh basil or Parmesan for topping
- salt & pepper to taste

Procedures:

- Cook pasta according to the directions for the package. Drain, toss with oil, and set aside to prevent sticking.
- Over medium heat, gently heat a large non-stick skillet. To the pan, add 1 tablespoon of butter. Sprinkle with 1/2

teaspoon salt and add the shrimp. Flip & cook until the shrimp is cooked. To keep warm, set aside and cover.
- Add the garlic and one tablespoon of the remaining butter. Add the corn and tomatoes; sauté for 1-2 minutes. Spinach added; sauté until wilted.
- Add the shrimp to the pan again. Add the remaining half of a teaspoon of salt and lemon juice. Add the cream and bring it to a low boil.
- Toss your sauce with the cooked pasta. As needed, add the reserved pasta water. Top with basil, Parmesan, salt, or black pepper, which is freshly cracked.

TOMATO SPINACH CHICKEN SPAGHETTI

Recipes:

- 1/4 cup of sun-dried tomatoes chopped, drained of oil
- Two tablespoons of olive oil drained from sun-dried tomatoes
- 1/2 lb of chicken boneless and skinless (preferably, boneless skinless thighs), chopped
- 1/4 teaspoon of salt
- 1/4 teaspoon of red pepper flakes
- 1/4 teaspoon of salt
- Four Roma tomatoes chopped
- 1/4 cup fresh basil leaves chopped
- 8 oz of spinach fresh
- Three garlic cloves chopped
- 8 oz of spaghetti pasta
- Three tablespoons of olive oil (use high-quality olive oil or oil from the sun-dried tomatoes jar)

Procedures:

- On medium-low heat, add the chopped sun-dried tomatoes and two tablespoons of the olive oil drained from the sun-dried tomatoes to a clean large skillet.

- Add a chicken chopped. I have used and prefer to use boneless skinless chicken thighs, but you can also use chopped chicken breast.
- Add red pepper flakes & salt over all of the ingredients in the clean skillet.
- Gently cook on medium heat until the chicken is cooked through & no longer pink, about up to five minutes.
- Top the chicken skillet with chopped tomatoes, chopped fresh basil leaves, fresh spinach, and chopped garlic. Cook for about 3-5 minutes on a medium heat until the spinach wilts a little, and the tomatoes release some of their juices. Withdraw from the heat.
- Taste, and, if required, add more salt to taste. Cover the lid and keep the heat off.
- According to package instructions, cook pasta until al dente.
- Drain the skillet with the chicken and vegetables and add the cooked and drained pasta.
- Reheat on low heat, mix well, add more seasonings, if desired (salt and pepper). Withdraw from the heat.
- At this point in time, when the vegetables & pasta are off heat, you can proceed to add more olive oil. It's voluntary but very tasty!

FENNEL SALAD WITH CUCUMBER AND DILL

Recipes:

- Two big fennel bulbs- trimmed and cored
- Three small Persian cucumbers
- 1/2 cup of fresh chopped dill
- 1/4 cup of white onion, thinly sliced (optional)
- ⅓ cup of olive oil
- Three tablespoons of lemon juice (Meyer lemon is nice, or sherry vinegar or, champagne, or red wine vinegar)
- pepper to taste
- kosher salt to taste

Procedures

- Halve the fennel bulbs and remove the hard core from them.
- Shave the fennel thinly using a mandolin and place it in a bowl (Or finely slice as thin as possible).
- Finely slice the mandolin with the cucumber and chop the dill. Slice onion finely.
- Add the olive oil, lemon, salt, and cracked pepper and place everything in a bowl. Before serving, leave to marinate in the fridge for 15 minutes.
- Taste, adjust the lemon and salt.

CABBAGE SALAD WITH CORN

Recipes:

- 1/2 medium of cabbage about 1 1/2 lb.
- ½ of English cucumber, sliced
- 1 cup of corn frozen and thawed or canned
- 1/3 cup of chopped dill
- 1 1/2 tbsp of vinegar
- 3 tbsp of olive oil
- 1/2 teaspoon of salt
- 1/2 teaspoon of pepper or to taste

Procedures:

- Start off by very thinly slicing the cabbage. If you have one, you can use a mandolin to help you slice it.
- In a large mixing bowl, place the sliced cabbage and add salt and pepper. Massaging the cabbage using your hands (as if you are kneading dough). This will soften and release some juices from the cabbage so that it becomes moist.
- Add all the remaining ingredients and mix well with each other. Just serve.

SPINACH AND SUN-DRIED TOMATO ZOODLES

Recipes:

- Six zucchinis
- Two tablespoons of olive oil, divided
- ½ cup of sun-dried tomatoes in olive oil
- One tablespoon of pine nuts
- ¼ teaspoon of red pepper flakes
- One garlic clove, minced
- 2 cups of baby spinach, roughly chopped
- Juice of a half lemon
- Freshly grated Parmesan cheese
- Fresh chopped basil

Procedures:

- Place the sun-dried tomatoes in a blender bowl and pulse until they are finely chopped. Transfer and set aside in a bowl.
- Create zucchini spaghetti using a spiralizer (always read the instructions as they vary by brand - I use this spiralizer). Make use of a regular vegetable peeler to vertically peel long, thin strips of zucchini if you do not have a spiralizer. This, like fettuccini, will form more of a broader "noodle" from the zucchini.

Heat one tablespoon of olive oil over medium to high heat in a large skillet. Add the zucchini noodles once hot and cook for about 2 to 3 minutes, until the zucchini noodles are tender, but some crunch is still retained.

- For about 3 minutes, let the noodles rest so that they can release all the moisture. Drain the leftover water from the pan & transfer the noodles to a colander.
- Wipe clean, heat the skillet over medium heat & add pine nuts. Cook & stir until it is lightly toasted, about 3 minutes. Transfer and set aside in a bowl.
- Heat the rest of the tablespoon of olive oil and add to the skillet the red flakes of pepper and garlic. Sautè for 1 minute over medium-high heat, until fragrant.
- Add spinach and cook for about one minute, until it is almost wilted.
- Then Add chopped sun-dried tomatoes, zoodles, & lemon juice. Stir until it is combined & heated through.
- Sprinkle with nuts, Parmesan cheese, pine & basil.

Serve and Enjoy!

CLASSIC POTATO PANCAKES

Recipes:

- Four large russet potatoes
- One medium onion
- Two egg
- 1/4 cup all-purpose flour
- salt, pepper
- vegetable oil for frying

Procedures:

- Peel and cube the potatoes and onion when using the food processor. Place the vegetables and process them for about 2 minutes in the food processor until the potatoes look "grated" and no lumps remain. Peel the potatoes and onion and grate when using the grater.
- Place a fine strainer or kitchen towel with the potato mixture and try to squeeze almost all of the liquid into a clean mixing bowl.
- Discard the fluid. After you pour the liquid out, you'll notice white powder on the bottom of the bowl. It's potato starch, and it provides the pancakes with texture, so you should keep it.

Return the mixture of potatoes to the bowl and add the eggs, flour, some salt, and pepper, and mix well.

- Heat some of the vegetable oil over medium heat in a large, non-stick skillet. Add a spoonful of the potato mixture and slightly spread it out. Fry on both sides for almost 2 to 3 minutes, until the pancakes are crispy and brown.
- On a paper towel, place the pancakes to absorb the excess oil and ENJOY!

ZUCCHINI NOODLES WITH AVOCADO SAUCE

Recipes:

- One zucchini
- 1 & 1/4 cup of basil (30 g)
- 1/3 cup of water (85 ml)
- 4 tbsp of pine nuts
- 2 tbsp of lemon juice
- One avocado
- 12 sliced cherry tomatoes

Procedures

- Proceed to make the zucchini noodles using a peeler or the Spiralizer.
- Then blend the rest of the ingredients (except the cherry tomatoes) in a blender until it becomes smooth.
- Combine the noodles, avocado sauce & cherry tomatoes in a clean mixing bowl.
- These avocado sauce and zucchini noodles are better fresh but can be stored in the fridge for up to 2 days.

EASY CREAMY CHICKEN PICCATA

Recipes:

- 1 Cup of Chicken Bone Broth
- 1 Lemon juiced
- ½ Cup of Coconut Cream blended before using
- ¼ Cup of Capers drained
- Lemon wedges to serve
- Freshly chopped herbs to garnish
- 1½ lbs. of Boneless, Skinless Chicken Breasts pounded to 1/2-inch thickness
- Sea salt & freshly ground black pepper
- ¼ Cup of Gluten-free Blend Flour
- 3 Tbsp of Olive Oil divided
- 4 Garlic Cloves minced
- 1 Small Onion chopped

Procedures

- On both sides, season the pounded chicken with a pinch of salt and pepper. In a clean, shallow bowl, place the flour in it.
- Gently heat two tablespoons of oil over medium heat in a large skillet. Bring up the chicken in the flour on both

- sides, working with one cutlet at a time. Shake off the excess flour & add it to the saucepan.
- Cook the chicken on each side for 4 minutes, or until it is cooked through and the coating is golden brown. Transfer to a plate the browned chicken, and set aside.
- Lower the heat to medium-low in the same pan and add the remaining tablespoon of oil, onions, and garlic. Sauté for 2-3 minutes until the onions are softened, stirring occasionally.
- Add the broth and lemon juice and use a silicone spatula to scrape the browned bits from the bottom of the pan. Raise the heat to a medium-high, & cook the mixture for 3 minutes, occasionally stirring, until reduced by half.
- Stir in the cream of the coconut and the capers, and place the chicken in the sauce. Simmer over low heat for up to 3 minutes or until thoroughly heated. Season with sea salt and black pepper to taste.
- Serve warm over sautéed cauliflower or cooked rice.

SWEET AND SOUR CUCUMBER NOODLES

Recipes:

- 3 teaspoons of fresh lemon or lime juice
- 3 TBSP of extra virgin olive oil
- 2 TBSP of white vinegar
- 1/4 tsp of salt plus extra, to taste
- 1/8 tsp of dill (fresh or dried)
- 1/8 tsp of garlic powder
- 1/2 tsp of fresh minced garlic
- 1/4-1/2 cup of fresh chopped cilantro plus extra to garnish
- 2 TBSP of honey
- 2 TBSP of rice vinegar
- One big English cucumber
- Toasted sesame seeds & chia seeds for topping

Procedures:

- Whisk everything together but the last three ingredients and pour over the noodles.
- To soak up all the yummy dressing or pop it in the fridge for later, let them sit at room temperature.
- Whisk the honey and rice vinegar together before serving and drizzle heartfully over the noodles.

- Garnish with a sprinkle of cilantro or chopped green onion with toasted sesame seeds and/or chia seeds.
- Crushed peanuts or cashews are also excellent! Based on what you have available as well as what you prefer taste/topping-wise, it is ridiculously simple to customize! Grab an English giant cucumber, a veggie peeler/spiral slicer, and go nuts!
- Serve for maximum flavor at room temperature.

ROASTED BROCCOLI QUINOA SALAD

Recipes:

- 1 cup dry quinoa
- 2 cups water (or veggie broth)
- ½ pound broccoli, cut into florets
- One sweet potato, chopped into ¼ – ½ inch chunks
- One can (15 oz) chickpeas
- One bunch laccinto kale, roughly chopped
- olive oil, as needed
- 1/3 cup fresh parsley
- 3 Tablespoons feta cheese
- juice from one lemon
- 1/2 Tablespoon apple cider vinegar
- Two teaspoons maple syrup
- 3 Tablespoons olive oil
- salt and ground pepper, to taste
- crushed red pepper, to taste (optional)

Procedures:

- Then bring the quinoa & water to a boil in a clean medium saucepan. Cover, reduce the heat to low, & simmer until the quinoa is tender or for 15 minutes. Remove from the heat & all to stand, covered, for up to 5 minutes. Use a fork to remove the lid and the fluff. To a large bowl, transfer the quinoa.

- To the quinoa, add roasted broccoli, spinach, and green onion. Drizzle it with fresh lemon juice & olive oil. Stir gently. Add the feta cheese, chopped pistachios, and season with salt and black pepper to taste. Just serve.

HONEY GARLIC ROASTED CARROTS

Recipes:

- 2 pounds of carrots cut into 3-inch pieces
- 1/2 cup of butter
- 2 tbsp of honey
- Four garlic cloves minced
- 1/2 tsp of salt
- 1/4 tsp of fresh ground pepper
- Freshly parsley

Procedures:

- Preheat the oven to 425°C
- Melt the butter in an oven-proof skillet. Add in honey & garlic and whisk until combined.
- Add in the carrots and coat with a toss.
- Bake in the oven until the carrots are fork-tender or for 25 minutes.
- Optional- To caramelize the carrots a bit, broil for 3-4 minutes.
- Sprinkle with parsley that has been chopped.

KALE SALAD

Recipes:

- 1 lb. of kale
- One large semi-sweet apple
- 1/3 cup of roasted almonds

Dressing Ingredients:

- 3 tbsp. of extra virgin olive oil
- 2 tbsp. of freshly squeezed lemon juice
- One garlic clove
- A half teaspoon of salt

Procedures

- Remove the kale stalks and discard them. Roll the kale into a bunch and thinly slice the leaves.
- In a clean large mixing bowl, gently place the kale leaves. Add the salt & massage the leaves until the kale starts to soften plus wilt, about 2-3 minutes.
- Add the kale with the olive oil, lemon juice, and garlic. Stir thoroughly and set aside.
- Peel the apple and core it. Dice it into small pieces & add them to the salad. Stir well, everything.
- In a serving bowl, transfer the salad and sprinkle the nuts on top. Just serve.

GARLIC HERB ROASTED POTATOES CARROTS AND GREEN BEANS

Recipes:

- 1 1/4 pounds of baby red potatoes (halved and larger ones quartered)
- 1 pound of medium carrots (scrubbed clean, cut into 2-inch pieces and thicker portions halved)
- Three tablespoons of olive oil (divided)
- One tablespoon of fresh thyme (minced)
- One tablespoon of fresh rosemary (minced)
- Salt
- freshly ground black pepper
- 12 ounces of green beans (ends trimmed, halved)
- 1 1/2 tablespoons of minced garlic (4 cloves)

Procedures

- Preheat the oven to 400°C. Toss potatoes, carrots with 2 1/2 tablespoons olive oil, thyme, rosemary in a large bowl & season with salt & pepper to taste. On a rimmed 18 by 13-inch baking clean sheet, spread. Roast for up to 20 minutes in a preheated oven.
- In a bowl, combine the green beans with the remaining 1/2 Tbsp of olive oil and lightly season with salt. Add other veggies to the baking sheet, add garlic and toss

everything and spread it into an even layer. Return to the oven & roast for up to 20 minutes until all the veggies are tender and slightly browned. Serve it hot.

ROASTED CAULIFLOWER STEAKS

Recipes:

- Two heads of cauliflower
- One teaspoon of kosher salt
- ½ teaspoon of black pepper
- ½ teaspoon of garlic powder
- ½ teaspoon of paprika
- ¼ cup of olive oil
- One teaspoon of chopped parsley

Procedures:

- Adjust the oven rack to the third position below. Preheat to 260oC (500oF)
- Remove the green outer leaves from the cauliflower head & trim the stem.
- Gently cut the cauliflower in half lengthwise through the center using a large knife.
- From each half, cut a one and half-inch-thick steak. Carefully cut one more steak from each of the cut sides of the head is large.
- Repeat with the other cauliflower head process. Trim any florets which are not linked to the stem. About 4 to 8 pieces in total should be there.

- On a rimmed baking sheet, put the cauliflower steaks.
- Mix the salt, pepper, garlic powder, and paprika together in a small bowl.
- Drizzle each side of each cauliflower steak with olive oil.
- Sprinkle the seasoning mixture evenly, about 1/4 teaspoon per side, on both sides of the cauliflower steaks.
- Close well the baking sheet tightly with a clean foil & bake for 5 minutes.
- Take the cauliflower off the foil and roast for 10 minutes.
- Flip the cauliflower steak gently and roast until both sides form a golden-brown crust, about 7 to 8 mins.
- Move to a serving dish & garnish with par filling.

HOT TURKEY AND CHEESE PARTY ROLLS

Recipes:

- 1 Stick of Butter Melted (½ cup)
- One 8 ounces tube of Crescent Roll Dough
- 12 to 16 Slices of Turkey (Deli Sliced)
- 12 to 14 slices of Colby Jack Cheese
- ¼ teaspoon of Garlic Powder
- 2 Tbsp. of Chopped Parsley
- 1 tsp. of Poppy Seed

Procedures:

- Roll out Crescent Roll Dough & press the diagonal seam together into four rectangle shapes.
- Put 3-4 slices of turkey and cheese on each rectangle.
- Roll each rectangle up (roll from one short side to the next short side) and gently press the seam together (You will have four rolls at this point).
- For a total of 12 rolls, slice each roll into three pieces.
- Spray cooking spray on a 9/13 baking dish
- Place rolls in a baking pan with 9/13
- Combine the butter, garlic powder, and parsley in a small bowl.
- Crescent Rolls Brush over and Sprinkle with Poppy Seed

- Bake for up to 15 minutes, at 350 degrees, until it just starts to turn brown.

CONCLUSION

Thank you for reading my book on the Mayr diets, and I hope you found it very interesting and explanatory.

Made in the USA
Monee, IL
04 June 2021